KAMA SUTRA

MASTER THE ART OF KAMA SUTRA LOVE MAKING

Judith Singh

© 2017

© Copyright 2017 by Judith Singh - All rights reserved.

The following eBook is reproduced below with the goal of providing information that is as accurate and as reliable as possible. Regardless, purchasing this eBook can be seen as consent to the fact that both the publisher and the author of this book are in no way experts on the topics discussed within, and that any recommendations or suggestions made herein are for entertainment purposes only. Professionals should be consulted as needed before undertaking any of the action endorsed herein.

This declaration is deemed fair and valid by both the American Bar Association and the Committee of Publishers Association and is legally binding throughout the United States.

Furthermore, the transmission, duplication or reproduction of any of the following work, including precise information, will be considered an illegal act, irrespective whether it is done electronically or in print. The legality extends to creating a secondary or tertiary copy of the work or a recorded copy and is only allowed with express written consent of the Publisher. All additional rights are reserved.

The information in the following pages is broadly considered to be a truthful and accurate account of facts, and as such any inattention, use or misuse of the information in question by the reader will render any resulting actions solely under their purview.

There are no scenarios in which the publisher or the original author of this work can be in any fashion deemed liable for any hardship or damages that may befall them after undertaking information described herein.

Additionally, the information found on the following pages is intended for informational purposes only and should thus be considered, universal. As befitting its nature, the information presented is without assurance regarding its continued validity or interim quality. Trademarks that mentioned are done without written consent and can in no way be considered an endorsement from the trademark holder.

TABLE OF CONTENTS

Introduction: What the Kama Sutra Can Teach You 1

Why was the Kama Sutra Created? 2

The True Meaning of the Kama Sutra: 3

What this Book will Give you: 3

Description 5

Chapter 1: The History and Philosophy of the Kama Sutra 7

The Kama Sutra, an Evolutionary Work: 7

Eastern Understanding of Humans and the Whole: 9

Kama Sutra in History: 11

Is the Kama Sutra a Manual for Marriage? 13

What is the Ananga-Ranga? 14

Bringing Old Wisdom to a New World: 16

Chapter 2: The Kama Sutra and Kissing 19

The Kissing Sutra: 19

Chapter 3: Beginner Sex Positions 27

Easy Positions to Try at Home: 27

Chapter 4: Intermediate Sex Positions 31

Intermediate Positions to Try at Home: 31

Chapter 5: Advanced Sex Positions 36

Chapter 6: The Importance of Foreplay 41

Pleasing the Female Partner: 41

How to Improve your Skills in the Bedroom: 42

Preparation in the Kama Sutra: Fellatio 45

Kama Sutra Cunnilingus Techniques to Please your Partner: 49

Cunnilingus and Fellatio, the Crow Position: 52

Chapter 7: Tantric Sex Techniques 53

Rituals for Pleasure and Power: 53

Tips for Preparing yourself for Tantra: 55

Tantric Sex isn't just about Orgasms: 61

The Tantric Yoni Massage: 62

Five Techniques for the Yoni Massage: 64

Tantric Edging: 66

Sacred Sexuality and the Penis: 67

Performing the Penis Lingam Massage: 70

Get lots of Practice: 77

Conclusion..**79**

Introduction: What the Kama Sutra Can Teach You

Congratulations on downloading your personal copy of *Kama Sutra: Master the Art of Kama Sutra Love Making.* Thank you for doing so.

Ancient sages in India created the Kama Sutra based on the famous Vedas. The first version of this book, which translates to the "rules of love" is said to be written by Shiva's companion, Nandi. This book is still preserved in the modern day and widely referenced, used and appreciated by people of multiple cultures across the world.

The Kama Sutra, in its original form, was one of a few different Indian texts that discussed the aims and goals of life. These philosophies state that life needs three different types of activity. These are the activity to assure that it will survive, activity to realize its continuation, and to create rules of behavior. It also states three aims or necessities in life, which are material goods, erotic practices, and morality or rules to govern behavior. These together all make sure that the human species will continue.

WHY WAS THE KAMA SUTRA CREATED?

It's believed that in the beginning, man and woman were created by Brahma to stand for creation and duality. At this point, he laid down some rules for humans to live. Although a lot of texts talk about the three activities of life mentioned above, the Kama Sutra is intended to cover Kama (desire) because many teachers ignored and overlooked this crucial element.

Each book of the Kama Sutra explains different ways a woman and a woman can come together that helps them develop in a positive way. It also talks about specific ways that people (especially men) should handle certain situations.

The True Meaning of the Kama Sutra:

Fulfillment of desire and love was overlooked very often by Indian culture, and sometimes even shunned. So when the Kama Sutra was written, the book was specifically aimed at the people who wished to understand the desire (Kama) and how to apply it to their specific situations. This isn't only sexual desire but desire itself apart from that.

Desire has two sides to it, negative and positive. Positive desire has a healthy and self-affirming nature, and negative desire is damaging to both us and others. So, the Kama Sutra provides the outline for having healthy, loving relationships with the people around us, not only sexually, but outside of that. It also teaches how to differentiate our personal wishes and desires.

What this Book will Give you:

The true meaning of this book is to find contentment in relationships and creating conditions with love with the people around us. This book will focus mostly on the sexual expressions of desire and how to use this to reach fulfillment both with yourself and the one you're in partnership with.

There are plenty of books on this subject on the market, thanks again for choosing this one! Every effort was made to ensure it is full of as much useful information as possible. Please enjoy!

DESCRIPTION

We've all heard of the Kama Sutra, but how is this book still relevant to us in the modern age of relationships? In *Kama Sutra: Master the Art of Kama Sutra Love Making,* you will learn:

- **The History and Philosophy of the Book:** The Kama Sutra doesn't have a single author and was even forgotten for a few centuries until it was rediscovered again. Learn about these topics and more in chapter one of this book.

- **Kissing in the Kama Sutra:** Kissing is often forgotten as an act of foreplay and as a way to enhance sexual intercourse. In chapter two, you will learn all about the different types of kisses, what they mean, and how to use them to enhance your sexual excitement with your partner.

- **Beginner, Intermediate, and Advanced:** This book will cover a chapter each on beginner, intermediate, and advanced sex positions.

- **Foreplay in the Kama Sutra:** In what ways can you effectively pleasure your partner, whether they are a male or female? What's the importance of foreplay in a sexual relationship? Learn about this in chapter six.
- **Tantric Sex Techniques:** Tantric sex is a way to spice up your relationship in the bedroom. This involves breathing techniques, massage, and more. The last chapter of this book will cover these topics in detail so you can put them to use.

There's a reason why the Kama Sutra is still well-known after all these years. It's more relevant than ever now, so don't hesitate to learn about it!

Chapter 1: The History and Philosophy of the Kama Sutra

Kama involves enjoying certain objects using your five senses; smelling, tasting, seeing, feeling, and hearing, using your mind but assisted by your soul. This involves a certain contact between the object and the sensing organ, and Kama refers to the pleasure that comes from this contact.

The Kama Sutra, an Evolutionary Work:

Ancient Indians were good evolutionists, as evolution shows that survival and sex are the most important forces behind our survival as a species. In addition, the Kama Sutra is an evolutionary book since it promotes the skills need to become evolved enough to have intimate, healthy relations with others. What other qualities does the Kama Sutra have?

- **Non-Pornographic:** Contrary to what some think, the Kama Sutra isn't a pornographic book. Actually, it's an image of the way a refined and civilized citizen should live, including the pleasures of life, eroticism, and love.

- **Cultivating Intimacy:** The book doesn't just instruct someone to be a good spouse, but to be intelligent, beautiful, sexual, refined, understanding, playful, skillful, and more. This ancient text also discusses the importance of cultivating intimacy and sensual moods and for males to understand their more feminine nature. The book also expresses the importance of attention to touch, drink, food, music, lighting, and more before sex begins.

- **Intimacy Within:** Our modern world is a stressful, busy place. It takes effort and time to create a sensual, beautiful environment and to build ourselves. A lot of people, especially females, don't have the sexual relationship they want to have. The Kama Sutra also called the Book of

Love or Art of Love, guides us toward an inner intimacy, both with the universe and others.

- When it comes to real intimacy, fewer inhibitions, true sharing of power, and freedom happens. The Kama Sutra isn't always popular or politically correct. However, the book is always thought-provoking, sensible, wild, creative, and even amusing. If you have an interest in sex on a historical level instead of just the act of sex, the Kama Sutra is worth reading. This book, however, is meant to give you the gist of the book without needing to read through the whole ancient text.

EASTERN UNDERSTANDING OF HUMANS AND THE WHOLE:

You can find a lot of wisdom from ancient ideas, especially old Indian Philosophy. Perhaps one of the greatest lessons is, the Eastern believe that everything is interconnected and that humans are connected to the whole universe. As we realize that connection, we find peace, guidance, and fulfillment for life.

- **Western Science:** Indians in ancient times were close to having an awareness of the true reality, even though they didn't understand matter. Western science, which is formulated on Time, Space, Forces, and Particles, hasn't ever truly grasped the interconnection of the universe.
- **Recent Discoveries:** Recent scientific discoveries on matter and its Wave Structure, along with Space's properties, gives a logical answer to the ancient Indian understanding of the universe.
- Hopefully, you will enjoy what you learn from this book and start to practice not just the Kama Sutra's techniques and wisdom, but the wisdom of knowing that you are connected to the whole.

KAMA SUTRA IN HISTORY:

The Book of Love (or Kama Sutra) is more complicated than just a book of complicated sex positions. Rather, it's a manual for a true, good existence. This book is the world's most ancient book about sexual living and pleasure. The book does not have one single author. It was compiled originally by an Indian sage from the north of the country in some part of the 3rd century. The sage claimed that he was a monk (and thus, celibate), and used the act of compiling sexual information to contemplate God and as a way to meditate.

- **A Significant Historical Text:** The Kama Sutra was written in complicated Sanskrit but is the only textual recording that survives from that particular period of Indian history. Scholarly circles have widely referred to the Kama Sutra in an attempt to understand the social norms of that time period. The book title means the pleasure treatise and is meant to give thorough advice to women and men alike.

- **Learning the Art of Pleasure:** One of the main ideas of the Kama Sutra is that for happy marriages, both women and men should learn about the art of pleasure, both mental and physical. Within the book is social ideas, society, sexual union, getting a wife, how to attract other people, and more. It also talks about how men can win women over, how women can win men over, the states of mind a woman goes through, and why women may reject men.
- **Types of People:** When it comes to choosing a partner, the book advises people to either follow childhood friends or fellow students. In addition, it gives charts that talk about female and male body types and how compatible they may be with the body of their lover. Different types of sexual intercourse, oral sex, biting, scratching, kissing, and embracing is also discussed. The book also talks about dealing with extramarital relationships.

Lastly, if the information within the text on winning love isn't enough, the last chapter of the Book of Love has recipes for foods, powders, and tonics that could attract other potential lovers to yourself.

Is the Kama Sutra a Manual for Marriage?

Some think of the Kama Sutra as a manual for a happy marriage, but it's very different from the dutiful and monogamous marriage manuals from the West. One of the Kama Sutra's main figures is a courtesan who must learn and master arts of coercing and pleasing her man. In addition, the book puts attention on pleasuring the woman. It says that a man who cannot provide pleasure to his woman has to accept that she may look for pleasure elsewhere.

The Rediscovery of the Kama Sutra:

The Kama Sutra was the original sexuality study but was also inaccessible and complex due to the language it was written in.

For that reason, the book became obscure for many, many centuries. Sanskrit scholars in ancient India didn't bother to look much into it. Around late into the 19th century, the book finally began resuming its popularity in India's textual traditions. This resurgence happened around the 1870s. Sir Richard Burton, a noted Arabic translator, and linguist worked with some collaborators, both British and Indian, on translating it.

Due to this man's persistence in bringing the book to the Western world, and the fascination people overseas and in India had in it, the book has now become as popular as it is today including all of its translations.

WHAT IS THE ANANGA-RANGA?

The Ananga-Ranga is a book from the 15th century that is the updated format of the famous Kama Sutra. This book is written in a language that is far easier to understand than the version before it, using a more accessible version of Sanskrit. Due to this, the Ananga-Ranga, for some years, was considered the more popular text for discovering information about sex and pleasure than the Kama Sutra. Ladakhana, a nobleman, was the one who commissioned the Ananga-Ranga to be written for a monarch of the Lodi Dynasty.

Wide Distribution:

This group of people was among the ruling class that presided over northern India in the times before it was replaced by the Mughal Dynasty. The author of this book was called Kalyanamalla, a poet, who consulted the Kama Sutra heavily while he prepared this text. He wrote in an easier to understand the style of Sanskrit, so the book was widely distributed throughout the Muslim empires of the age.

Different Versions:

The Ananga-Ranga appeared in many different languages, including Urdu, Persian, and Arabic. Starting with a dedication for the patron of the text, Ladakhana, this book has descriptive advice for spouses, regarding both their sexual and social activities. This starts with some descriptions of the female body, along with the erogenous zones, body type classifications, their potential pleasures, and centers of passion.

Compatibility and classification of females and males by the size of their genitals are looked at in multiple scenarios and combinations. A lot of scholars think that the author existed in a society that was more sexist than writers of the earlier versions since he didn't provide advice for the female's pleasure. Other texts described and endorsed methods for this, such as advising using fingers. The title Ananga-Ranga can be translated to the Hindu Art of Love or the Stage of the Bodiless One.

BRINGING OLD WISDOM TO A NEW WORLD:

Under colonial rule and its romanticism, Europeans looked for Eastern texts for the purpose of bringing the wisdom within them to the new world. But since the Ananga-Ranga had

Orientalist engagement, this led the book to become decreasingly relevant, as the Kama Sutra became more popular. Burton had experiences with life in India from being a part of the military that was stationed there, and he became fascinated with Oriental sex practices. This fascination, paired with his desire to bring this knowledge back home, led him to Sanskrit texts about the topic.

How the Kama Sutra Regained Relevance:

Due to the state of the popularity of the book at the time, according to specialists of Sanskrit, perhaps it was most logical that this text became Burton's top choice. When he looked over the translations of the text, though, Burton noticed a lot of the references involved in the translation. He then considered that the Kama Sutra was more relevant and valuable and requested to find a copy. Since it had been relatively neglected for centuries, the book at that time was only available in portions. It had to be re-collected from sources around India.

As soon as it was translated to the English language, it grew in popularity and scholars in India cast the Ananga-Ranga aside in favor of the Kama Sutra. It's because of all this that the book is now commonly heard of and referenced, even in the English-speaking Western world.

Chapter 2: The Kama Sutra and Kissing

Contrary to what many people believe, the Kama Sutra is not only about sexual interactions. Kissing is a very important aspect of a romantic partnership. This chapter will cover some tried and true techniques for kissing.

The Kissing Sutra:

Kissing is the initial activity a couple will take in the direction of a sexual relationship. This activity is a crucial part of their time together and must be enjoyed equally by both parties. Otherwise, a lack of chemistry with kissing can end the relationship fast. Within the Kama Sutra, many different kisses are described. When you learn to recognize these moments with your partner, you may perfect and fine-tune them to reach the fullest potential of enjoyment for you both.

Kissing is an important aspect of foreplay and should never be forsaken or overlooked when sex is in the near future. In addition, kissing is important during the actual act of intercourse. Apart from the literal penetration, kissing is among the most affectionate and personal activities the couple can engage in. Let's look at a few different types of kissing.

- **A Straight Kiss:** Also known as the direct kiss, this involves the two lovers' lips being brought together directly in a straightforward way. It is among the more exciting kisses in the book of the Kama Sutra since the couple is face to face and completely immersed in kissing, sucking, and licking the lips of the other, at times with tongue play involved. This is one surefire signal that there is something steamy coming up next.
- **The Askew or Bent Kiss:** Considered one of the more romantic types of kisses, this is ideal for slower sex and is very charged with emotion. This type of kiss happens when thelovers' heads bend forward. When this bending

occurs, the kiss happens. This is one of the more popular types of kisses and is also among the more common. The bent angle of the heads allows for each tongue to enter the other's mouth in a deeper way. This kiss is a great way to begin a passionate session or encounter.

- **The Clasping Kiss:** This is when either the female or male takes the other's lips between their own, clasping on. This is an odd type of kiss that most don't do and a woman can only take this type of kiss from a clean-shaven man without a mustache. This kiss has given by someone looking to try something different with their partner.

- **A Turned Kiss:** This occurs when one person turns the other's face toward them, usually with their hand or by holding their chin. This kiss is very personal and shows a specific intent when the partner directs the other's face toward them.

- **The Tongue Fighting Kiss:** If during a kiss, one partner uses their tongue to touch the other's teeth or palate, this is called the tongue fighting kiss. The majority of people will instantly recognize what this kiss means since it's so passionate and usually means that foreplay or heated sex is coming up soon. This type of kiss also can and should be used to intensify sexual activity.

- **A Love-kindling Kiss:** When the female peers at her lover's face as he sleeps and gives it a kiss to show that she wishes to have sex, this is called a love-kindling kiss. A male will learn to recognize this look on his woman's face after some time with her.

- **The Unexpected Kiss:** It's a good idea to randomly give your partner an unexpected kiss when you're together or when they are engaged in something else. This helps to nurture the growing relationship and show them that you care.

- **A Pressure Kiss:** This type of kiss might seem aggressive but is enjoyable to many people. This involves keeping the lips and mouth of the other person closed and biting. This should only be done sparingly, so you don't cause pain to your partner. Keep in mind that not everyone will enjoy this type of kiss.

- **A Top Kiss:** When you share a kiss with your partner that leads to delicious feelings, this is a top kiss. This involves one partner using their teeth to take in their partner's top lip, while the other partner does the same thing to the other's bottom lip. This can be alternated with each person's tongue, leading to a progression of foreplay and added excitement.

- **Throbbing Kisses:** This is the sweeter and more tender of kisses and is known as a throbbing kiss. This involves one partner kissing their partner repeatedly across their mouth and is a classic way to demonstrate romance and love. When given by your lover, it's an instant way to feel special and valued.

- **A Contact Kiss:** This is perfect as a prelude for a steamy session of sex and involves two partners struggling to resist holding back their desire. One of the partners will then lightly touch the mouth of the other, in a provocative manner, using their lips to make intense, light contact. This should be very short and enticing for the other.

- **The Flame-igniting Kiss:** The book of the Kama Sutra involves an innocent-seeming kiss that is actually not very innocent at all. This is meant to ignite a flame in your partner and involves kissing the corner of their mouth. This will leave them unable to notice the hint that you want more from them.

- **The Distracting Kiss:** This kiss has a clear purpose that is obvious from what it's called. This kiss is meant to draw your partner's attraction and doesn't only have to take place in the mouth. In addition, it can be used on the chest, neck ear, face, or other erogenous zones of either partner.

- **An Eyelash Kiss:** This is a very sweet, loving, and intimate action and happens when you caress your lover's mouth using your eyelashes. This is especially good for those who have long or thick eyelashes.

- **The Finger Kiss:** This type of kiss is tantalizing and exciting from start to finish. One lover will put their first finger in the mouth of the other, remove it, then brush the finger across their lover's mouth. The gesture hints at the invitation or allusion to oral sex later on. This can also be done during sex to spice things up and intensify the session.

- **The Parting or Farewell Kiss:** This is the kiss used for the classic goodbye and involves touching your lover's mouth with your fingers after kissing. This can be provocative in the right setting even though it's a simple gesture.

- **The Awakening Kiss:** This kiss is ideal for when your lover is sleeping, and you want to gently wake them up with a kiss on their temple or forehead. This can be done before having a nice breakfast together or before having sex before starting your day. Gestures such as this will keep you close to your partner.

- **The Kiss in Public:** This is a way to send others a clear message about your intimacy and relationship. This can be a kiss on the neck or hand, which states that you are willing to be perfectly open about what exists between you and your partner.

Kissing is a wonderful and enjoyable way to contact your partner. However, as we grow in age and think more about sex, kissing can be forgotten during sex. The ancient book of wisdom, the Kama Sutra, focuses intently on this type of contact and gives it great importance. The book states that when we unite our senses together, great emotions can be experienced.

Chapter 3: Beginner Sex Positions

The Kama Sutra book is a text from ancient India that was intended to help people (especially men) engage in happy, fulfilled marriages. Though a lot of people believe it's just a collection of pornographic images and advanced sex positions, there is only a single chapter out of seven that is completely about sex.

Easy Positions to Try at Home:

Modern versions of the old Kama Sutra teachings are popular because of the "equal congress" or mutual pleasure they advocate. The ones listed in this chapter will be suitable for beginners. Keep reading to get a useful summary of beginner Kama Sutra sex positions.

Intermediate Sex Position #1: The Pillar.

The woman and man, both unclothed, will kneel on the floor facing toward each other. The woman will then spread her thighs, showing herself to him. The male will then draw the woman closer to him so that she can sit on his thighs and guide his penis closer to her. The man needs to sit erect and embrace his partner in an intimate hug. This allows each partner to caress and kiss each other comfortably. Although this limits stimulation and doesn't allow for deep penetration, the caressing will still allow for a pleasurable and sensual experience together.

Intermediate Sex Position #2: The Goddess.

For this position, the male will sit down with his chest held straight. The woman will guide his penis into her vagina, sitting atop him with her legs wrapped around his body. She can move her hips back and forth as she sees fit, allowing for deep penetration and an intimate union. This position lets the partners kiss, and the man fully caress the woman. For the man, the stimulation is comparatively limited, making it very suitable for men who have a problem with premature ejaculation.

Intermediate Sex Position #3: The Indrani.

For this sex position, the female will lie back and bend her knees toward her chest. She is then able to pull her partner toward her body by grasping his hips or linking her hands behind his bottom. She may rest her legs in his underarms, controlling how close his torso gets to her body. This position will focus on the woman's beauty since her position makes her appear like a flower in bloom. In addition, this position is great for couples that have a man who is larger than necessary to satisfy the woman.

Intermediate Sex Position #4: The Mill.

This sex position is still simple and beginner-level but does require a bit of flexibility. For this move, the man must lie back while the woman kneels or squats above him, waiting to be entered. His penis will be used as her axis to spin upon. She can shift her legs over his chest, turning her body until she is reversed atop him. She can then switch back and forth as she sees fit. This changes the view for each partner and keeps things interesting.

Practice the positions listed above for a while until you feel comfortable with them and don't be afraid to add your own twists to them! Once you're comfortable with all of the beginner positions, it's time to move onto the intermediate level positions in the next chapter.

Chapter 4: Intermediate Sex Positions

Whether you hope to get a fast, short sex session in, or a longer, deeper penetration, the Kama Sutra book likely has a suitable position. If you're hoping to advance beyond the missionary position, the Kama Sutra has been guiding people into new positions for countless years. Although some of these might sound complicated, they won't be too hard to master if you're willing to practice!

Intermediate Positions to Try at Home:

If you're wanting to try out a specific position, having an excited and positive attitude will help a lot. This way, both partners will have a pleasurable and fun time no matter how it goes. It also helps to have a sense of humor. When you're ready to give it a shot, proceed.

Intermediate Sex Position #1: The Sammukha.

This position is relatively simple, and you might never have thought you'd try it. For this move, the woman will lean her body back up against the wall as she stands, spreading her thighs open as much as possible as you enter. This will lower the woman's body slightly, so if she is shorter, it's best for her to stand on top of an ottoman or stool. Men who are taller might have to kneel down if the woman is flexible. Though this will feel slightly awkward initially, it's very romantic and passionate due to the eye contact going on. Since the woman will be holding herself up against something, the positions offer amazingly deep penetration.

Intermediate Sex Position #2: The Janukurpara.

This intermediate move will likely call for some extra time at the gym, but the extra intimacy with your loved one will be well worth the effort! For this move, the man must lift the woman up, locking his elbows beneath her knees and holding onto her buttocks with his hands. She will then lock her arms around your neck to hold herself steady. This will allow for some eye contact, plenty of deep penetration, and offers the man a chance to look heroic and strong. A lot of these flexible positions let you brag and also offer you a lot of pleasure. This position can be your way to reward yourself for hitting the gym.

Intermediate Sex Position #3: The Piditaka.

Some people will soon learn that acrobatic or flexible doesn't always equal more pleasure. This position is laid-back, comfortable, and can be done at any time, even after you've just had an intense leg workout. The woman will lie back and put her knees up toward her face and chest, then rest her feet upon the man's chest while he kneels down before her. The man will keep his knees placed on both sides of her pelvis, then lift her body and hips onto his thighs while he penetrates.

The woman will feel tighter because her passage will be narrowed by the position of her legs. She may cross her feet or press her thighs in more to increase pressure on you both if that's what you desire. This sex position is ideal for couples who enjoy positions that offer female vulnerability. If you want to stay even truer to the Kama Sutra, the man can hold her feet close to his forehead and mouth, be showing devotion, humility, and romantic tenderness toward her.

Intermediate Sex Position #4: The Virsha.

This position isn't unusual, but most of us know it as the Reverse Cowgirl. This position is often used in porn movies and not as much by everyday couples. It involves the woman being on top, allowing her to feel in control, strong, and sexy while offering the man a view of her bottom. The male should lie back as she kneels or sits over him and faces his feet. She will then lean her body forward and lower her vagina onto his penis while grabbing his ankles.

Intermediate Sex Position #5: The Tripadam.

This position is perfect for a quick sex session because it lets you have fast, short fun but doesn't call for very deep penetration. Both partners will stand up and face toward each other. The man will place his hand under her knee, lifting it up, then enter into her as he stays standing up. This will be a challenge for couples who are very different heights, however.

This position turns the couple into a tripod. Standing positions offer a maximum flow of blood to the genital areas and other erogenous zones, increasing pleasure and work best for couples who are around a similar height or within a few inches of each other. The positions in this chapter shouldn't require too much fitness or effort, but when you're ready to really challenge yourself (and each other), it's time to move on to chapter seven.

Chapter 5: Advanced Sex Positions

Having sex that is too predictable and routine can ruin your relationship, particularly when you've been together for many years. This section will help you find ways to challenge each other and keep your bedroom interesting and fascinating. Let's look at some of them now. Keep in mind that if you can't do these right away, that's okay. This will just give you an excuse to get lots of practice!

Advanced Sex Position #1: Erotic V Shape.

For this position to work the way it's supposed to, some gym time may be required because it will wear your legs out! To do the erotic V shape position, use a table and have the woman sit at its edge. The man should then position his body to be in front of hers, bending his legs to enter her. She should place her arms around him at the neck with her legs up over his shoulders. The woman should lean back as he thrusts. At first, this will be very tiring until you build up your stamina more.

Advanced Sex Position #2: The Ape Position.

This position allows you to get animalistic with each other. You don't have to be a gymnast to make this move, but it helps to be very flexible. This one works as the man lies back with his knees pulled up toward his chest. The woman will then sit on his hips, having him enter her. She will prop herself up while sliding it in slowly. Be careful with this position. It allows for a great, deep penetration but can be a challenge.

Advanced Sex Position #3: Catherine Wheel Position.

For the Catherine Wheel Kama Sutra sex position, each partner should sit facing each other. Once they are in the right position, she can wrap her legs around his middle, allowing him to enter her. The man should then wrap his leg over her pelvis, keeping her pinned in place. Be careful for this so she can stay on balance and he doesn't get a fracture. The woman should hold her body up using both of her hands, and he can guide her hips, creating the ideal rhythm for both.

Advanced Sex Position #4: The Sex Bridge.

For this position, the male needs to be very flexible and able to do a bridge position and hold it for a length of time. This position will start with the man putting himself into that position, creating a bridge. The woman will then straddle his body, sitting on his penis. She should be careful not to rest her weight on her feet as this could hurt his testicles. Once you're in position, make sure he can support his weight, and the woman can do the movement as he stays held in place.

Advanced Sex Position #5: Dolphin Position.

For this position, strong back muscles are absolutely necessary.

Strengthen those back muscles, you're going to need them for The Dolphin. Lie on your back and arch your back while holding yourself up by the shoulders. Your thighs and hips should be raised toward the ceiling. Keep your head and neck flat. Your guy then slides in between your knees and lifts your hips while he's inside you. He slowly humps you while checking your pulse. Kidding.

Advanced Sex Position #6: Seduction.

If you (as the woman) don't feel very comfortable sitting on your knees, this one might be hard for you or will require some practice. If you have spry knees, however, try it out! Initially, the woman must begin sitting on her knees, leaning her body backward with her feet tucked underneath her buttocks. She will then raise her arms up over her head. The man needs to lie on the woman with his legs straight, shimmying his body until he enters her, then the fun can start!

Advanced Sex Position #7: Plow Position.

This position will have the woman start off in front of the bed on her knees. The man then must help her to lift her body up onto the bed's edge, and she will also use her elbows to aid this motion. The woman should then straighten her legs out completely as the man holds her body up, stepping between her open legs. She will lift her hips as he enters her. Picture a tractor for this position and start moving as you two see fit.

These advanced positions may take some practice or time at the gym, but don't get discouraged. If they are too difficult for you, it's time to go back to the basics. In the next chapter, we will cover the importance of foreplay as well as some specific instructions and guidelines you can use to get the most out of this crucial part of sex.

Chapter 6: The Importance of Foreplay

The book of the Kama Sutra isn't only about sexual intercourse and also focuses heavily on the necessity of foreplay. This chapter will focus on cunnilingus and fellatio, which (when done right) will prepare each partner for a fun-filled night of sex. Many individuals, and women, in particular, enjoy oral sex a lot. Becoming accustomed to the Kama Sutra's subtle arts will help you elevate your stamina and bedroom performance, pleasing your partner and becoming closer to them over time.

Pleasing the Female Partner:

This chapter might be especially useful for the men who are not as inclined toward loving or passion, or who fall asleep as soon as they have climaxed. The Kama Sutra can help men to realize that the female's needs will differ greatly from theirs. This information is important to consider if you are aiming to get a fulfilled relationship that will last a long time.

- **No Selfishness:** Quality love making has no room for selfishness and instead is about respecting and learning about what your lover needs and wants to feel satisfied, then make sure you give it to them.
- **Long Term Love:** Relationships that understand this crucial step will have plenty of passion-filled evenings and will last the test of time. Who doesn't wish for that with their love?

How to Improve your Skills in the Bedroom:

In order to have the best bedroom skills possible, observe the following rules. These techniques for Kama Sutra foreplay will give you more intense sex sessions and help please your partner.

- **Always Care for the Other:** Before you get to touch in a sexual way, the book of the Kama Sutra will instruct you to engage in some important activities first. This can involve feeding each other fruits or pastries, drinking champagne or wine, lying outdoors together or having a nice conversation. The emotional connection you share here is very important to how successful the foreplay methods will go for each of you.

- **Fully Embrace:** The joining of two physical bodies, naked or clothed, shows significant feelings that exist between each of them. This will let you receive full benefits of building up toward the sex act. Blend the four essential components of the Kama Sutra for bodily connection: pressing, piercing, rubbing, and touching. When you are lying together, keep in mind that the woman's forehead, breasts, genitals, and thighs are the key areas to focus on for sexual desire.

- **Woman in Charge:** The Kama Sutra outlines roles for women and men, but the woman should be encouraged to let out some aggression sexually and even assume the dominant role during foreplay. This will create a new, exciting dynamic and increase intensity for both parties.

- **Light Biting:** In the Kama Sutra, light biting is recommended. When you do bite the other focus on the nipples, earlobes, and lower lips. This will create a love quarrel that is playful, romantic and helps to bring about sexual satisfaction over the long term. You can integrate biting into disrobing and use your teeth to take the other's clothes from their body.

- **Using the Nails:** Before doing this, make sure your hands and nails have been cleaned. During extreme passion, such as before sex or in an intense foreplay moment, the nails can be used to mark each other's bodies in an affectionate gesture.

Preparation in the Kama Sutra: Fellatio.

Oral sex can be used to prepare both parties for some intense intercourse. Thanks to the Kama Sutra, this chapter is full of some useful tricks and tips to improve the fellatio experience for your male partner. Keep in mind that quality fellatio relies on good rhythm and technique. Try out different rhythms and styles as you change pressure, speed, and depth.

The Touching Step:

When the woman holds the penis with her hands, making an "O" with her lips and then touching them to the tip while moving her face in a circular motion, this is known as Nimitta. This step is a great way to start for a woman who is unsure of what to do while giving oral sex.

The Nominal Congress Step:

Next, as the woman holds the penis in her mouth, moving her lips, this is known as nominal congress. This technique is mild, simple, and a great way to get acquainted with the act of giving oral sex to the man. This technique is not vigorous and instead relies on gentle motions of the tongue and lips around the penis tip.

Gentle Biting:

The next step involves the female holding the head of his penis in her palm, tightly clamping her lips around his shaft. She can do this on the side of the shaft, then on its other side, making sure her lips are completely protecting and covering her teeth. To put this another way, the head should be gripped in her fingers as her tongue and lips caress the length and shaft. This is a less intense way to start out fellatio.

Bahiha-Samdansha:

For this technique, the woman will bring the man's penis into her lips gently, kissing and pressing it gently while pulling the skin softly. This method is similar to the final step of his penis being withdrawn and taken into her mouth. The woman will give the penis gentle kisses after withdrawing it from the lips. Then, she can let his head completely slide in and out of her lips and mouth, firmly pressing the shaft in between her top and bottom lip. She can hold onto it momentarily before allowing it to slide out completely.

Fellatio Kissing:

The woman will then take his penis into her hand as she rounds her lips and fiercely kisses the whole length. She can suck the skin similar to the way she would suck his lip during a kiss. Good fellatio isn't only about fitting the whole penis into the mouth but about exploring it all with the tongue and lips to add variation.

Rubbing the Penis:

The next technique involves flicking the tongue over the penis, pointing it and running it repeatedly over the sensitive tip. This is an aggressive move but can also feel extremely erotic due to the sensitivity of the penis head. The woman should be sure not to use too much pain or pressure since this could cause discomfort.

Communication is key, and the woman should make sure that what she is doing doesn't hurt if she isn't sure.

Amrachushita:

Now, in a state of passion, the woman will bring his penis into her mouth deeply, sucking and pulling on it in a vigorous manner. This will bring him to a climax. Since this is a vigorous motion, the woman should be careful not to make too much noise since this can be off-putting. Putting some music on during sex is a good way to cover up noises if you are worried about them. It can also help to set a nice mood for sex.

Sangara, Swallowing the Penis up:

As soon as the woman senses his orgasm impending, she should suck and swallow the entire penis up, working on it with her tongue and lips. Whether or not the man should ejaculate inside her mouth should be up to the woman, and this should be discussed before you engage in this act. An agreement will prevent any unhappy accidents or misunderstandings.

Kama Sutra Cunnilingus Techniques to Please your Partner:

Good oral sex is an important part of making sure the woman is satisfied with the relationship. Follow these techniques, and she will be most pleased.

A Quivering Kiss:

These are instructions for the man:

Using your fingertips very delicately and gently, slowly pinch her arched lips together, kissing them as you should kiss her lips. This technique is strange but can be great if done the right way. Pinch the labia gently together so that they form a mouth and then give gentle kisses to it.

Circular Tongue Motions:

Next, the male can spread her labia open using his nose, allowing his tongue to probe her vagina and his chin and lips to circle it slowly. Keep in mind that the woman's vagina is highly sensitive and that gentle motions are important. The man should make sure he shaves his face so that there is reduced irritation for her.

The Massage of the Tongue:

Before proceeding, the man should allow his tongue to rest at the entrance of her vagina and then enter into it with his tongue. He should always keep therhythm in mind, switching up rhythms, pressure, and speed and mixing up the area he focuses on. In addition to this, he should pay attention to her reactions and stick to one area if she seems to like it.

Clitoris Sucking:

The next step involves the male fastening his lips against hers and kissing it deeply, sucking the clitoris and nibbling her gently. Her clitoris is the most sensitive part of her vagina and can be the quickest way to bring her to orgasm. Remember that communication is key and the male should ask his partner what she likes best, whether it's licking, circles, fast, or slow. He should find out for sure rather than just guessing what she prefers.

Skillful Rotating:

Next, the man should cup her buttocks, lifting her gently while he slithers his tongue down, skillfully rotating at the entrance of her vagina. Her entrance is a very sensitive spot that can produce immense pleasure for her if gently stimulated. The male should move his tongue in a circular motion, switching directions every so often to stimulate her area.

Hand Stirring:

The male should now stir her thighs at the root as she uses her own hands to hold them apart. The woman should help the male to give her the most pleasure by telling him what she desires and opening her thighs wide.

Hard Sucking:

Next, the male should pick his lover up and place her on a sofa, putting her feet on his shoulders as he clasps her at the waist. Then he can suck at her vagina hard and stir his tongue over her entire vagina. Keep in mind that sex shouldn't only occur in the sleeping room, and you can experiment all over the home to spice things up. You can use couches or high tables for easy access to each other's genitals.

CUNNILINGUS AND FELLATIO, THE CROW POSITION:

Also known as the "69," this position allows both lovers to pleasure each other at the same time. The pair of lovers must lie down next to each other with their heads facing opposite directions, kissing each other's genitals using the above techniques. This position is the most erotic choice for partner's giving oral sex to each other since they can share the sensations at the same time.

Chapter 7: Tantric Sex Techniques

Using the term tantric sex with your new date might intimidate them as much as it intrigues them. To a lot of people, tantric sex seems unique, exciting, and possibly more interesting than standard sex techniques. However, not many people actually realize that tantric sex is. In cultures throughout the world, sex is thought of as just a recreational activity. Tantric sex, on the other hand, is the old Eastern practice of spirituality intended to join feminine and masculine energies and to expand consciousness into the whole.

Rituals for Pleasure and Power:

Tantric sex is considered an old method for attaining both psychic power and sexual pleasure. Tantric sex enables participants to get to new heights of desire, pleasure, and to use their sexual energy for creativity and guidance in other areas of their lives.

- **Using the Power of Sexual Focus:** In sexual involvement, people are at their most intense concentration both consciously and subconsciously. Tantra allows you to carry that focus into the rest of your life, instead of keeping it to just sex.
- **Higher Pleasure:** In learning about tantric sex, the involved rituals allow you to have sex more, last longer in bed, and reach higher levels of pleasure than you used to. The more often you engage in sexual activity, the more powerfully and quickly this energy will replenish. With tantric sex, your faculties (including the emotional, mental, and physical) are all brought into high stimulation so that you can control them and reach higher pleasure levels.
- **Free from Hypocrisy:** Apart from its spiritual foundations, what about tantric sex is different from the attitude of sex we have in the West? Tantric sex is free

from hypocrisy and control and can present a path to an enlightened mindset.

TIPS FOR PREPARING YOURSELF FOR TANTRA:

Tantric sex is beyond what the average person enjoys in sex and must be approached with both an open mind and the right attitude and mindset. Here are some steps to help you in this process.

1. Prepare the Area:

Get the bedroom or other room you will be using for tantric sex ready with soft bedding and comfortable pillows. Use a lot of lit, but unscented candles in the room, in safe places of course. The lighting should be dim. You can put some wine or water within easy reach for you and your partner to drink from during your sex session. It might be helpful to keep some fruit or snacks nearby to stay energized. You can use a scented oil diffuser if you wish.

2. Prepare your Mind and Body:

This experience must be approached with your heart and mind completely open. If there is something in this process that makes you feel uneasy, you don't have to do it. However, when possible, try to move past this discomfort. Feelings of discomfort in sexual situations are usually the result of shame and during this practice, try to stay curious and playful in order to stay open to new types of pleasure.

- **Bathing or Showering:** Take a bath or shower with your lover or by yourself to prepare, but don't engage in any sexual touch yet. Face each other as you shower or bathe and then do some light stretching to get rid of anxiety or stress before you begin.

- **How to Dress:** For this, you should dress in nonrestrictive and comfortable clothes, such as a loose shirt, shorts, lingerie, or underwear. This can be done in the nude, too, but since you are trying to build sexual energy up from scratch, starting clothed is advised.

3. **Start Building the Energy Up:**

After you bathe, shower, and stretch. Sit across from your partner in a comfortable position. You can cross your legs or even place your legs over your partner's, allowing your erogenous zones to be closer to your lover's. The male can sit in a cross-legged position with the woman facing him and sit on his legs.

- **Eye Contact:** Gaze into the other's eyes for a while. This might feel awkward initially but make sure you keep looking until you feel more comfortable. There aren't any rules for how long to do it for.

- **Establish Comfort:** As soon as you get into a comfortable mindset, you've established the goal of a connection. This is the exact connection that is required for the enjoyment of tantric sex practices. Keep eye contact as you follow these steps.

4. Take Deep Breaths:

The next step involves breathing with your partner. Slow your breathing down and sync up your inhalations and exhalations, trying to breathe together while maintaining your eye contact. You may put your hand on your lover's chest if you wish to feel their breaths.

- **Sharing Loving Statements:** As soon as your breathing and eye contact is fully in sync, you can use words to further connect to each other. You can list what you love about each other or what you like about what they do. Go back and forth and make sure you're honest.

- **Light Touching:** Slowly and lightly move your hands over the body of your lover to wake up their nerves while keeping eye contact. You may tease and excite them by bringing your fingertips close to their erotic zones without touching them directly.

5. Tantric Kissing:

At this stage, you should practice some tantric kissing with the mouth open slightly and touching very lightly. Synchronize and share your breaths as you breathe in and out together. This can then lead you into a sensual, slow, soft kiss.

6. Full Body Massage:

For the next step, you and your partner can exchange full body massages. The one receiving the massage should start facing down as their partner massages non-erogenous areas for a few minutes at a time, then moves onto sexual areas. You can use your hands for this, or other objects if you wish to increase stimulation. As soon as you have massaged them all the way face down, ask them to flip over so you can get the other part of them. This massage isn't about reaching orgasm, so don't focus too much on sexual stimulation.

7. Tantric Sex:

The last step of this tantric practice is the sex itself. On the other hand, you can also lie together in a blissful, relaxed state of mind. Intercourse shouldn't be the main goal of this experience and is just one possibility. If and when you do decide to engage in intercourse, go slowly and pick the position that brings you into the greatest connection together.

- **Position Choices:** Preferably, you should choose a position that lets you look each other in the eyes the entire time. Most importantly, you shouldn't lose awareness during the act of sex. Instead, stay grounded and focused in the present, letting energy build inside of yourself.
- **No Rules for Time:** There isn't any rule for how long you can do this. This should be about letting pleasure unfold in whatever ways come naturally while staying as connected as possible to each other.

Tantric sex is an inspiring idea of sacred sex, which is lost to many Americans and people of the Western world. It involves approaching body parts, especially the vagina, from a mindset of worship. The Sanskrit word for vagina (yoni) translates loosely to "sacred space." Tantric philosophy encourages people to approach this body part with utmost respect and love. The massage of this area is meant to honor the female, to explore her sacredness, and to give her pleasure in a selfless gesture.

TANTRIC SEX ISN'T JUST ABOUT ORGASMS:

Tantric sex is never about having orgasms. It's all about attempting to heighten pleasure and to possibly create multiple orgasms throughout the entire experience. This can be done by yourself or with your lover, by itself or as a prelude to sex. This practice is especially beneficial to females who have trouble with climaxing.

THE TANTRIC YONI MASSAGE:

This type of massage will let the man explore the woman's body in a loving and sensual manner and can help females get to multiple orgasms. This massage can heal those who have gone through some kind of trauma sexually in the past. This is because this massage is centered on giving to the female, allowing her to feel honored, worshiped, cherished, and fully loved. Here are the steps for the tantric yoni massage.

1. Get Prepared:

As mentioned with the tantric sex steps above, when you begin this new practice, start with your heart and mind open and free from judgment of yourself or your partner. The woman should lie back comfortably and have a pillow underneath her pelvis, with her knees bent, feet on the floor. Have some nice smelling massage oil nearby.

2. **Connect through Breathing:**

This practice involves breathing, just as the previous one does. Breathwork matters a lot for anything involving Tantra. For this step, you should use the Bliss Breath, which involves inhaling as you tighten your throat, causing a whispering noise.

- **Breathing Guidelines:** Breathe out, releasing the same noise, and continue these breaths as slowly as you can, keeping them audible. This will help you get grounded within yourself instead of in your mind, spreading the energy of the climax within your bodies.
- **Spreading the Energy:** The woman should remember not to have her energy solely focused in your clitoris, but rather should try to spread it out across her whole being.

3. **Get Warmed up:**

Although stimulating the clitoris is awesome as sex foreplay, a tantric breast or body massage will be better for preparing for a yoni massage. This will build arousal while relaxing both partners.

Begin with your massage oil on the woman's stomach, massaging gently in that area. The stomach is usually overlooked on a woman but can feel good due to the nerve endings there. Massage her on the lower abdomen, between her breasts, and across her ribcage. As soon as her body starts responding, you can circle her breasts without touching her nipples. As soon as she starts to respond, even more, you can tease her nipples, lightly pinching, stroking, and alternating the pressure applied.

FIVE TECHNIQUES FOR THE YONI MASSAGE:

As soon as the woman's body is warmed up with the massage mentioned above, it's time to move onto the yoni massage next.

Make Circles:

This technique involves circling her clitoris using your fingertip, gently stimulating her arousal. You can use small and large circles, alternating pressure and intensity.

Pulling and Pushing:

The next technique involves pressing down on her clitoris as you stroke with small pull and push motions. Slide your fingertip along her clitoris's shaft, stimulating both sides. Pay attention to her reactions, since some women will have more sensitivity on one side than the other.

Rolling and Tugging:

In order to gently tug on her clitoris, pull it from her vagina as you grasp its sides and move it side to side. This can also be done a little lower on her lips. Your strokes should vary and go from the lips to the clitoris, then back down. In order to make the rolling motion on her clitoris, begin by holding it and rolling between your first finger and thumb.

Clitoris Tapping:

The clitoris can also be tapped using a finger or two. Simply tap this part of her using various rhythms and speeds until you notice what she seems to like the most.

Massaging her G-Spot:

In order to discover where your lover's G-spot is, make a curved shape with your two fingers, slipping them into her vagina. The G-spot will be a squishy lump somewhere behind her clitoris, and this can be massaged by gently stroking it. Use slow and fast strokes, alternating between them. You may also touch her clit at the same time or put some pressure above her pubic bone. Try to mix up the steps listed above, switching between them while also touching her nipples and G-spot.

TANTRIC EDGING:

Edging is a method that involves going to the edge of a climax repeatedly. As soon as your body is about to orgasm, you should pull away and slow down, then build it again in order to create many different waves. As your body is cooling down, your hand can be placed over the heart (or your partner's heart) to help your body stay in a grounded, connected place. This will help spread loving energy, and sexual energy can be built up again from here, then again slowed down, and so on. The longer this stage of foreplay is stretched out, the higher the pleasure will go.

SACRED SEXUALITY AND THE PENIS:

A huge portion of the concept of sacred sexuality is figuring out how to appreciate and love your man's penis, instead of being intimidated by it. The lingam massage in this chapter will first focus on the man doing it himself, then the man receiving the massage. This can be done alone or as a lead up to sex with a partner. A lot of women aren't completely comfortable with penises. If this applies to you or your partner, think about what negative experiences or impressions may have led you to feel this way.

In tantric sex, we are connecting with our lover personally, while also connecting to the universe through our lover's body. The lingam massage is one method for doing this. The lingam massage is basically a fancy term for giving your partner a handjob. But you do it with more desire, care, respect, and thoughtfulness to bring about unselfish pleasure and love for your lover. It's unlike a typical hand job in that it doesn't just involve the penis, but also the prostate, perineum, and testicles.

- **The Wand of Light:** Lingam means wand of light in Sanskrit. When it comes to Tantric practice, the lingam should be approached with respect and love, just as the yoni is approached, as discussed in the previous section of this chapter. When the partner is brought to pleasure using the wand of light, both parties are filled with light and energy in a conscious, aware energy exchange of pleasure swapping.

- **Honoring the Male:** The lingam massage will honor your man and can be done to give him truly, selfless pleasure. In addition, a lot of chi or sexual energy exists inside a man's penis. When you can learn to stimulate this energy, it has a profoundly powerful impact and effect. When people visit India, they will see statues representing the Shiva lingam. For a lot of people in that culture, this is meant to stand for meditation. However, for tantric practitioners, the depictions carry a secret and hidden meaning. The powerful energy of God exists not just in a man's body, but directly in his penis. This is the representation of masculine energy and essence in one area.

For sex to be truly sacred, the man's penis and body must be approached as a religious temple, with his penis being the pinnacle of holiness. This process shouldn't just be about a single orgasm but about heightening pleasure and possibly bringing multipleorgasms about during the massage session.

PERFORMING THE PENIS LINGAM MASSAGE:

Some men may wish to use this practice to cultivate energy and as a way to masturbate. If that's the case, just follow the directions here on yourself.

1. Relaxation:

For this stage, the male must lie backwards or sit in a way that is most comfortable for him. Some men may prefer to have a pillow under their heads or pelvic region. The male should bend his knees slightly with his legs spread, allowing his genitalia to be fully exposed. Remind the man to take deep breaths so he can fully relax as much as possible.

2. Breathing:

Breathing is the key ingredient in Tantra and is what truly separates it from ordinary sex that most people have. When the man is receiving his lingam massage, make sure both partners are engaging in the Bliss Breath mentioned earlier. This will help the woman receive the pleasure and arousal energy coming from him, and send him energy of love as she breathes out. This way of breathing offers three important advantages:

- A deeper appreciation and understanding of meditation, worship, and mindfulness during the massage session.
- A deeper understanding of empathy toward the male's feelings and thoughts.
- A heightened level of intuition sexually, helping the woman become more aware of what he wishes for, without the need of asking.

Remind your partner to take deep breaths throughout this practice. Before the massage begins, tune into each other's beings and minds by doing the Bliss Breathing in sync. Just breathing simultaneously will help you both get relaxed and feel into each other more. As the woman massages the man, she should remind him to relax, breathe deeply, and open himself up to all of the positive sensations and energies available.

3. **Massage with Lubrication:**

For this, you will just massage around the penis to start with, using the massage oil you prefer to use. Then you can oil up the penis and testicles. Begin sliding both hands along the thighs before you get to his penis, which will further relax him. You can give him compliments about him as you touch him.

- **Testicle Massage:** The next step involves moving onto his testicles and slowly, gently massaging them. You can slightly pull on them or even use your nails very softly. Cup his testicles in your palms, gently fondling them in a loving manner.

- **Surrounding Areas:** Next, massage around the penis and testicles, such as the inner thighs, front pubic bone, and the taint (between the anus and testicles). Make sure you're careful with his testicles since men are very different with what they prefer. Some guys will be ticklish and not like this area touched, while others will love it. Always ask if you aren't sure!

4. **The Shaft Massage:**

As soon as the areas surrounding the penis have been teased and he is in a state of desire, you can move onto the main attraction, his shaft. Use a varied grip, switching between light and hard touches, varying your sequences between twisting or just moving up and down in a straight motion. You can mix up this action, using two hands, then one hand. As you use a single hand, switch between the left and the right, so your hand doesn't get tired.

- **Varying Speed:** Begin slowly here and build the tempo up to something faster, then move back to slow movements. As you go along, vary methods, rhythm, speed, and the pressure of your hand and hands. Move them differently to keep it interesting.
- **Variety:** Alternate the strokes you use to begin at the bottom then working to the top of the penis. As you reach

the head, you can keep moving up and down or twist, starting at the bottom and stop at the top. Variety is what you should be going for at this stage.

- **The Two-handed Method:** If you decide to use both hands, this can be done in a few varieties. You can use both of your hands to hold in with your fingers all pointing the same direction, or use both hands to move simultaneously. Make sure you use plenty of oil to create a pleasant gliding, smooth sensation. Or you can use the bottom hand to make straight motions as the top one makes a twisting or swirling motion towards the penis tip.

5. **Hold off the Orgasm:**

You shouldn't allow him to orgasm yet. Instead, your goal should be to keep him right on the climactic edge. At this point, he may wish to come because he will be very excited and worked up. If you've been noticing his movements, moaning, and breathing, it should be easy to predict whether or not he's close to coming. Once you notice him at that point, slow down and pull back, reminding him to breathe deeply and enjoy the edge of the climax. His hardness might vary from semi-hard to very hard, which is normal and expected at this stage.

6. External Stimulation:

Next, you can stimulate his external spot from the outside. This is his prostate, the gland between his penis and bladder, which is about the size of a walnut. When it's properly stimulated, it can feel great for him. This can be accessed from the inside (by putting your finger into his anus) or from the outside by massaging his body in the right place.

- **Begin with the External:** For a guy who doesn't have experience with this, it's best to start outside. In order to locate this area of him, search for a slight indentation between his anus and testicles and gentle press. Make sure you are moving slow and listening to his reactions.
- **Massage:** As soon as you find the area, you can massage it using your knuckles or fingers. Gently press in, back off,

then press again. You may also utilize a massage motion of circular movements. If you're massaging a very hairy man, make sure you use oil.

7. **Internal Stimulation:**

Find out if your partner is interested in an internal prostate massage. If it turns out he is, he will need to be loosened up with oil. Begin by rubbing the outer area of his anus, using a gentle, smooth, slow motion with your fingers. Make sure you don't insert your finger without asking if he's ready.

- **Using enough Oil:** Once he's ready, ensure that your fingers and his anus are properly oiled. Ensure that your nails have been clipped recently, then start with just a fingertip. Move it back and forth to get him relaxed.

- **Insert deeper:** As soon as he is more relaxed, you may go deeper with your fingertip. Note that the prostate is located between two and three inches inside, close to the rectum's anterior wall. As soon as you've done this, you may caress the prostate by moving up and down or side to side. Let him tell you what feels best.

This type of massage can be difficult to perform using just the fingers, so some couples buy toys for this purpose. In order to bring the massage to an end, you may let your partner orgasm and then move onto sex, if he's ready. Remember that the sex should never just be about orgasms and that you should take your time, make lots of eye contact, and always remember to focus on the breath and breathe together.

GET LOTS OF PRACTICE:

Tantric sex is all about getting as much practice as possible with your partner, and this will bring you both closer together. Make sure your partner is interested in doing this, and even have him or her read this chapter with you, so you can work on it together and get very good at it. Once you're open to this world of tantric sex, the possibilities are endless! And most importantly, always remember to have fun together.

Conclusion

Thank you for reading *Kama Sutra: Master the Art of Kama Sutra Love Making*. Hopefully, you enjoyed it and learned a lot from this book. The Kama Sutra isn't just full of guidelines for how to have a fulfilling and loving sexual relationship, but also how to enjoy life and be a great person.

Many people are at a loss for how to spice up their relationship or marriage, but now you have the tools to make it happen. Don't hesitate to share this book with your partner, as well, so you two are on the same page.

Lastly, if you enjoyed this book, please leave it a positive review on Amazon! Thank you and good luck on your sexual and relationship related journeys.

www.ingramcontent.com/pod-product-compliance
Lightning Source LLC
Chambersburg PA
CBHW071752080526
44588CB00013B/2224